Your Perfect Day

A Mindful Wedding Planning Guide
for a Stress-Free Celebration

Claudia Marcela Chavarro
Licensed Mental Health Counselor

CKBooks Publishing

ISBN: 978-1-949085-85-3 (paperback)
978-1-949085-86-0 (ebook)

Claudia's Wedding Planner: Avec Moi Events and Design
Photography: Kaity Brawley

CKBooks Publishing
PO Box 214
New Glarus, WI, 53574
ckbookspublishing.com

To my husband, Paul, who did everything he could to make our wedding day a dream come true. I hope we can remember this special day for the rest of our lives, especially during tough times.

Table of Contents

Acknowledgment

I would like to thank my beautiful baby girl, Marcela Grace. Her sweetness motivated me to finish this project, which I started while I was pregnant with her. I will forever be grateful for her and the joy she brings to my life. I love you, my sweet girl.

Preface

One of the most anticipated events in every couple's journey is their wedding day. While the engagement period holds significant memories, it quickly transitions into a time of busy wedding planning. With so much to arrange and coordinate, it's only natural for couples to strive for perfection in every detail, whether it's the delicious cake, beautiful decorations, guest list, or attire.

In *Your Perfect Day: A Mindful Wedding Planning Guide for a Stress-Free Celebration*, I share my entire outlook on the prospect of marriage. I highlight important factors such as self care, reducing stress, avoiding conflicts by communicating effectively, and making smart decisions when planning an event.

I emphasize the importance of setting boundaries with family members when it comes to planning and how you can have healthy conversations while avoiding conflicts.

I've included my own experience of celebrating my big day during the Covid-19 pandemic. But my main message is that the wedding is more about the couple feeling fulfilled and happy than anything else.

Toward the end of the book, I explain what should be avoided before the big day and provide efficient tips about what to expect.

In addition to all the pre-wedding and wedding day preparations, I also cover post-wedding blues, something that is often over-looked because it's not normalized to feel sadness after your special event is over.

This book is intended to help everyone, but especially people who face some anxiety before any major event in their life.

Chapter 1

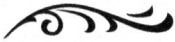

Utilizing Wedding Planners, Family, and Friends

The thought of getting married can evoke a range of emotions. You might feel joyful about sharing your life with your soulmate, thrilled to embark on a new journey together, nostalgic about bidding farewell to your single life, and anxious as you plan your dream wedding. Weddings can be a hassle if not done right. You have so much to do, and even if you take a lot of time planning, there's always a chance of something going wrong.

Right after my engagement, I was excited to start planning and making decisions to make our wedding day memorable. However, I soon realized how overwhelming it all was, which emphasized the importance of seeking assistance from a planner and relying on the valuable support of my loved ones. There were countless things to consider: What venue should we choose? How many guests can we invite? And so on.

During this planning time, there's no substitute for additional help, be it from an experienced wedding planner or the caring assistance of close friends and family. Hiring a professional planner can ensure that your big day goes smoothly, while also providing unique skills and insights for designing and organizing your special day. Involving family members and friends can further support your vision. Their personal touch can add warmth and familiarity to the event. Delegating tasks to people you trust will help reduce stress and allow you to spend the day having fun, dancing, eating, and catching up with your loved ones.

It's not uncommon for couples to feel anxious and stressed about planning a wedding. With so much to do and so many decisions to make, it can feel overwhelming and difficult to manage. That's why having help from others can be such an invaluable asset.

After the engagement, make a budget with your significant other and start consulting wedding planners, if this is the route you want to take. I contacted many but hired the one I connected with the most. I reviewed how organized their website was and how quickly they responded to my request.

Once you have found a suitable wedding planner with whom you feel comfortable, start your preparations. As you plan, consider how others can assist with the various aspects of the wedding. The collective efforts of those around you can enhance each element of your wedding.

Selecting dependable vendors also plays a vital role in the planning process. Your loved ones can be supportive, but they may not be able to assist with every-thing on your big day. Having a team of trusted vendors to handle last-minute details can be beneficial, allowing you to enjoy the day with family and friends fully.

A wedding planner will know every vendor there is, can advise you on which ones to book, and can direct everyone on your special day. When my wedding planner gave me my wedding day timeline, I realized how much she had orchestrated and how much she had worked during the previous eight months. She had gone through every single detail, big and small, and presented an impeccable layout of the entire wedding day. From the moment we were getting ready to the moment the first dance began, she had accounted for all the vendors and parts of the day. Each step of the process was laid out in a timeline that allowed us to stay on track and ensured nothing but a beautifully organized day.

After selecting the venue and vendors for your wedding, it's a good idea to start searching for your dress and suits. It can be helpful to decide on your preferred style beforehand and then make appointments at different boutiques. Searching for the perfect gown that fits just right and gives off the exact style you want to display on your special day can be stressful. But don't worry—this is where trusting your instincts comes into play. You are the best judge of what makes you feel confident and beautiful. Listen to your gut. It can help you find the perfect wedding dress that truly resonates with your style.

The same goes for the bridesmaids' dresses. Being diligent and careful with reviewing delivery dates and contracts is key to handling any unexpected problem that may arise on the supplier's end. For instance, the bridesmaids' boutique I visited initially proposed a delivery date one week before the wedding. At first, I didn't think anything of it, but reviewing the contract carefully allowed us to negotiate an earlier delivery date, ensuring everyone had time to make necessary alterations.

To ensure you look and feel your best on your wedding day, it is important to schedule a hair and makeup trial with your stylist beforehand. This will give you the opportunity to try out your desired look and make any necessary adjustments. Remember, feeling confident and comfortable with your appearance will reflect in your photos and overall happiness on your special day.

My engagement pictures were taken twice because the first makeup and photography session was a disaster. The photographer never told me my bra was showing in most of my photos, and the makeup artist overdid my makeup! I don't wear heavy makeup, so having a lot of makeup made me look completely different, which was not the idea. I wanted to look my best self, not like someone else. So, witnessing my dilemma, my planner led me to meet a more suitable makeup artist and a more professional photography team.

Designing and sending out invitations is a crucial step in wedding planning that can quickly become overwhelming if you do it alone. Delivering the right message and diligently keeping track of who received the invitation and who has RSVP'd is essential. Maintaining an organized system can make this process much simpler. I initially had a few errors on my guest list. However, through careful double-checking and cross-referencing, I was able to catch all the mistakes, ensuring everyone's names and addresses were in order.

Due to the pandemic, my invitations got delayed by the US Postal Service. Fortunately, I had sent save-the-dates and created a website with all the information. My planner also contacted everyone by email and sent them a digitally designed invitation. Everyone had the information on time, and the hard copies arrived just a few weeks after expected.

At a wedding, you will have all sorts of guests: family, friends, colleagues, acquaintances, and so on. To ensure that everyone is taken care of and not neglected during the festivities, it is wise to plan ahead and keep track of their needs. On the day of my wedding, it was extremely helpful to have a planner and venue coordinator around to direct us. They knew when and where everyone had to be for photos, events, and more.

Since we are on the subject of guests, let's also talk about seating charts. They are critical because they determine who will be up front, closest to you, and who you'll have in the back. Designing these charts properly takes time, which you may not have. A wedding planner can create your seating chart according to your preferences and choices, considering how you want the tables set. This will help ensure that your guests are seated appropriately and comfortably, allowing for conversations between certain individuals, such as family members or close friends. Once these seating arrangements are final, it is easy to decide who sits where.

Having photographers at a wedding is a deal breaker as they capture all the significant and heartfelt moments of the special day. For my wedding, we carefully selected a team who could capture the day exactly how I had imagined it. Before choosing a photographer, it's important to take some time to compare and select a photographer that fits your preferences and budget.

The bridal bouquet and flowers are one of the most important elements of any wedding, adding beauty, style, and color to the bride's look. The flower arrangement should complement your dress, and it should also coordinate with the overall wedding theme. I held the most beautiful flowers, which complemented my dress and also went well with my wedding décor.

A honeymoon is perfect for newlywed couples to start their life together. It's an opportunity to relax, spend quality time with each other, and explore a new destination. Although it may not be a part of the wedding day, you should still dedicate time to planning your post-wedding trip if you intend to take one. Take some time to look up reviews and compare the prices of the places you have in mind. We were lucky enough to have a family member help plan ours. If you have a family member who is a travel agent, don't be afraid to ask for help. My husband's aunt did a fabulous job showing us resort options and planning our trip.

There are many more details that I could go over with you, like selecting a band or an officiant, which are equally vital to a wedding. But this chapter should have given you a clear idea of how elaborate a wedding can be and why it is crucial to allow others to help. Feeling supported will take a lot of pressure off your shoulders.

In my experience, hiring a wedding planner was very helpful because I was new to the area and didn't have much support from family and friends leading up to the big day. However, if you have family in town that can help, most planners offer different packages based on your specific needs. While hiring a planner is an additional expense, they can help you save money in other areas. Weddings can be stressful for both the bride and groom. Having the support of professionals and loved ones is the best way to ensure a healthy and enjoyable experience.

Chapter 2

~~~

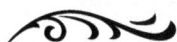

Navigating Through Critical Decisions

In the exhilarating journey of planning your wedding, decisions take center stage, enticing you to make choices that will shape your special day into a cherished memory. Like a delicate dance, each decision can transform your vision into reality, weaving together a tapestry of love, joy, and celebration.

Planning a wedding involves carefully considering various aspects such as the wedding dress, decorations, menu, music, and more. Feel free to confidently make decisions that align with your vision and values while navigating the challenges of compromise and balance.

While it's important to consider the advice of vendors, planners, and those you trust when deciding parts of your wedding, I would advise you to remain true to your vision as much as possible. I received some recommendations that didn't align with what I had in mind, but by being honest about my preferences, others were able to better understand the type of celebration I wanted. The following are a few pointers that can help you smooth out your planning progress:

- Understand your budget.
- Stay focused on your vision.
- Compare vendors to see who meets your needs.
- Don't give much attention to social media if it's overwhelming.
- Limit your research and set a deadline for your final decisions.
- Rank your options before signing contracts.
- Trust those who are helping you.
- Communicate well with your future spouse.

Understanding your budget is a top priority, and deciding everything according to that is even more critical. An event as big as a wedding needs a set budget to cover everything without running short on funds. One of the biggest mistakes people make, when it comes to wedding budgeting, is over-spending. It can be easy to get caught up in all the excitement and lose sight of what you can actually afford without going into debt.

It is easier to make decisions when you know your budget. For instance, when you have less capital, you might not get the venue of your dreams or have a destination wedding, which rules out some options. However, you can get creative and explore venues close to your hometown that could also offer a beautiful experience.

Aftcr understanding what you can and cannot do, reflect on what you would like. Even when some options are out, you still have many from which to choose. My wedding planner always used to say, "Tell me what you want, and I will get creative with it."

Every person has their idea of how their wedding should be. It's important to stay true to your own ideas and not get too sidetracked by the suggestions of others. For example, I didn't want a sit-down rehearsal dinner simply because we would have had more than ten toddlers. I imagined doing something more relaxed where the kids could play and the adults could still enjoy each other. Even though having a rehearsal dinner was very traditional, we chose to do something different because of our circumstances.

After choosing your vendors, you still need to make more decisions. Social media can be helpful in wedding planning but it can also complicate your decision-making process by offering you too many alternatives. If you're struggling to decide, it's best to take a break from your phone.

Scrolling through hundreds of social media photos with incredible floral arrangements or beautiful dresses will only make it harder for you to focus on the details you're currently considering. I tried on so many wedding dresses, they all looked the same in my mind at the end of my search. Ultimately, I chose the first one I tried on that felt represented me the best. Let your wedding planner or a friend help you limit your options and go for what you want most within those options. Rank your options based on what best represents your vision. Make a pros and cons list, and spend some time considering the benefits and downsides of the alternatives you have.

Setting deadlines helped me a lot. When I took too long to decide, I would give myself a deadline and move on. After spending months looking at pink shoes online and falling asleep with the phone in my hand, I realized that my decision-making strategies needed to change. Meeting contract deadlines and setting personal ones are crucial in reducing stress and achieving a smooth decision-making process. The following are some helpful tips to assist you in establishing your deadlines:

Understand Your Timeline

Start by identifying your timeline until your wedding day. The time estimate will assist you in determining when particular decisions must be finalized.

Prioritize

Not all decisions have equal weight or urgency. The venue, for example, must be decided much earlier than what kind of flowers to have on the tables. Identify the most critical decisions and assign them early deadlines.

Break Down Big Decisions

Larger decisions, like the guest list or venue, can be daunting. Break these into smaller tasks (e.g., researching venues, scheduling visits, final selection) and set deadlines for each.

Use a Planner or Digital Tools

Use a wedding planner or digital tools like apps and calendars to help keep track of your deadlines. Set reminders to ensure you remember everything.

Be Realistic

Be mindful of your other commitments and personal limits while setting deadlines. The wedding planning process should be joyful, not overly stressful.

Delegate

Remember, you don't have to do everything yourself. If it's too overwhelming, delegate tasks to your partner, family, or a wedding planner, if you have one.

Buffer Time

Allow for some wiggle room. Things may not always go according to plan, so having buffer time before each deadline can be beneficial.

Decisiveness

Once you've reached a deadline, trust your instinct and decide. Avoiding prolonged choices will help to reduce stress and keep the planning on track.

Remember, these are your deadlines. Be

flexible and adjust them as necessary based on your circumstances and the specifics of your wedding. It's all about maintaining balance and ensuring the planning process is enjoyable. I had to make some last-minute changes to the table assignments. Although it was stressful, I was able to accommodate a few additional RSVPs, which I was happy about.

At times, due to stress, conflicts arise between couples during the planning of their wedding. Don't worry. I'll guide you through some circumstances you can try to avoid. You may also want to consider completing a premarital counseling course. If you need help finding a certified premarital counselor in your area, you can search online or ask your clergyperson for a recommendation.

Money and sticking to a budget can become a constant debate when planning a wedding. Take some time to talk with your future spouse and decide what you can realistically afford. Emotions can take over and cloud the decisions you make in this area. Make sure you are not going to need to take out a large loan to cover the cost of something you can do without. One day is not worth years of debt. Bad financial decisions can make your wedding day become a day you don't want to remember.

At the start of planning, my husband and I became too enthusiastic about certain aspects and had to remove some things towards the end. We were able to communicate and agree on things we could mutually do without and tried to keep those items that were meaningful to us. My husband is a big food guy and didn't want to let go of his menu selection, and I didn't let go of my Hora Loca, a popular tradition in Latin America. (Hora Loca is Spanish for "the crazy hour.") We did decide to get rid of the ice cream stations and compromised on doing a very simple welcome social/rehearsal dinner. We discussed our nonnegotiables and worked around them.

Sit down together, communicate assertively, listen to each other, and work out the details of your wedding. Weddings are all about working together and communicating with each other. They mark the beginning of a permanent life change, which is why it is crucial to have these conversations.

Tips on communicating assertively:

- Voice your opinions in a respectful tone.
- Listen to each other and take turns talking.

- Negotiate and compromise.
- Try to make decisions with a clear mind, not after a long day of work.
- If the conversation is not going anywhere, take a break and talk about the planning at some other point.
- Respect each other's reality.
- Express your needs and feelings.
- Use "I" statements if needed. For example, "I feel frustrated when you avoid talking about the budget for the band because we have a deadline."

Chapter 3

~✦~

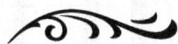

Setting Boundaries

Boundaries are essential in both our personal and professional lives. They help us stay true to ourselves and assert our autonomy in relation to others. In particular, healthy boundaries with family members and friends are essential for maintaining relationships and developing mutual respect. In this chapter, we're going to focus specifically on how to keep healthy boundaries with your family and friends.

In marriage, boundaries are equally important. They protect you from harmful outside influences and help you strengthen and maintain a healthy relationship with your partner. Planning your wedding together can allow you to share your personal preferences and limitations with your future spouse. Communicate these preferences and boundaries with love and care as differences arise.

It's natural to encounter various opinions and distractions from others. Boundaries can help you stay focused on your vision for your special day. The steps below can help you maintain calm as you make decisions about dates, menus, dress codes, etc.

Define Your Vision

Clearly articulate and align your shared vision for the wedding. Discuss your desires, preferences, and overall theme.

Communicate Your Boundaries

Share your intentions and boundaries with your loved ones and friends. Let them know that while you appreciate their input, you and your partner ultimately have the final say in the decision-making process. Many people asked me to change my wedding date. At some point, I had to decide based on our plans.

Select a Trusted Inner Circle

Surround yourselves with a select group of close friends and family members who genuinely support and understand your vision. These individuals will act as your sounding board and provide constructive feedback, ensuring your choices align with your vision.

Prioritize Open Communication

Maintain open lines of communication with your partner throughout the planning journey. Regularly discuss any concerns, changes, challenges, or suggestions that arise. Doing this will enable you to address any conflicts promptly and ensure that you both remain on the same page.

Stay Focused on What Matters

Amidst the noise and potential distractions, remind yourselves of the core elements that truly matter to you both. Keep your focus on the significance of your commitment, the love you share, and the joyous celebration of your union.

Embrace Flexibility

Recognize that unexpected changes or compromises may arise. Be open to adjusting your plans when necessary while staying true to the essence of your vision.

Take Time for Self-Care

Remember to prioritize self-care and quality time together. Take breaks from the planning process to relax, rejuvenate, and enjoy each other's company.

It can be challenging to navigate wedding planning when family members disagree with some of your decisions. As a couple, it's always important to present a united front. Effective communication skills are crucial during this time. By assertively expressing your thoughts and feelings, you can navigate these situations without compromising your vision or relationships.

Here are some examples of how you can express some of your boundaries:

Decisions About the Wedding Venue

"We appreciate your suggestion, but we've spent some time discussing and decided that [chosen venue] is the best fit for us. We really hope you'll come to love it as much as we do."

Disagreement About the Guest List

"We understand you'd like us to invite more people, but we've decided to have a smaller, more intimate wedding. We hope you understand and respect our wishes."

Budget Issues

"We really appreciate your input, but we're trying to stick to our budget. It's important for us to start our married life without unnecessary financial stress."

Interference with Wedding Dress/Suit Choice

"We value your opinion, but what we wear on our big day should ultimately be our decision. We've chosen outfits that we feel comfortable and happy in."

Dispute Over the Wedding Date

"We've considered all the possible dates and believe that [chosen date] works best for us. We understand it might not be perfect for everyone, but we hope you can make it."

Family Traditions or Religious Customs

"We understand this tradition is important to you, but we want our wedding to reflect our personal beliefs and preferences. We hope you can respect our choice."

Involvement in Planning Details

"We know you're trying to help, but we've decided to handle the wedding planning ourselves/with our wedding planner. We'll be sure to ask for your help if we need it."

Remember, when saying no, always be respectful and clear about your decisions. It's your wedding, and it should reflect you as a couple.

Although establishing and maintaining boundaries may not always be easy, especially with family. Clearly defining your limits and expectations is important to maintain a healthy balance between your own needs and the needs of others.

If you need help setting up boundaries, consider the following example. You can create your own based on your specific situation.

What is the boundary?

The couple will not change the wedding plans in response to someone threatening not to attend.

How can it be communicated?

"We understand your specific request and appreciate your input. However, our wedding plans are final, and we cannot accommodate that request. We hope you can still attend and celebrate this special day with us."

Why does the boundary need to be in place?

The boundary is in place to assert your autonomy and preserve the integrity of your wedding plans. It's important to prioritize your vision and make choices that align with your desires as a couple.

How long should this boundary be in place?

The boundary should remain in place until the wedding takes place. You can extend and modify the boundary if a similar situation arises after the wedding.

What if it doesn't work?

It's crucial to remain firm in your boundary while expressing empathy and understanding. Reiterate that you would love to have that family member present and emphasize the significance of their support. However, avoid sacrificing your happiness and values to appease their demands.

If the situation becomes difficult to navigate or causes significant distress, it can be helpful to seek the support of a therapist.

Remember that setting boundaries is about honoring your needs and creating an environment that promotes your emotional well-being. By asserting your choices and maintaining boundaries, you establish a precedent for future interactions and dynamics within your relationships.

It's important to consider how much involvement you want from your family. It can be uncomfortable to hear statements such as, "I'm paying for the dinner, so I get to give the speech." If your family members are contributing financially, make sure you establish clear boundaries. Will their contribution give them control over the menu or the speeches? If so, it might be best to cover the costs to ensure the celebration reflects your vision and creates lasting memories for you.

By openly communicating your expectations, discussing areas of potential compromise, and setting clear boundaries, you can navigate wedding planning discussions respectfully and constructively. Remember to express appreciation for their support while emphasizing your need to maintain certain elements that hold deep meaning for you and your partner. Discussing important matters through emails and texts can often lead to misunderstandings, which may cause valuable information to get lost. Having face-to-face or video conversations could help avoid stress and ensure clarity in communication.

Many brides are lucky to have supportive family and friends, but not all have this privilege. It's completely acceptable not to invite toxic family members and instead choose guests who will happily help and celebrate with you on your special day. Trust your instincts and make this decision together.

When considering those who genuinely want to be more involved, think about ways they can contribute. For example, my sister read a passage during the ceremony, and my brother gave the blessings at the reception. Additionally, my sister-in-law was thrilled to help coordinate the selection of bridesmaids' dresses and did a fantastic job. Their involvement made the day even more memorable.

Setting boundaries may sometimes leave you feeling overwhelmed, guilty, and confused, but having supportive individuals with whom you can share your feelings and thoughts can help ease these emotions. Practicing self-care activities like taking a yoga class, spending time with your partner, or meditating after a long day can also help.

Chapter 4

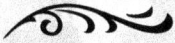

Planning Your Wedding
in Stressful Circumstances

Planning a wedding in the middle of a pandemic or under other circumstances that are out of your control adds extra stress on the bride and groom. I had to plan my wedding in the middle of a global pandemic. Horrifying? Well, not quite. It would have been troublesome if it had been during the peak time of the lockdown. Luckily for us, our wedding was one year after the pandemic started. Things had started to settle down a bit, and businesses had figured out safe new ways to operate. There were still many restrictions, but fortunately we were not among those who had to cancel their entire event. This chapter focuses on ways to cope with stress if unfortunate events like a pandemic or family emergency surfaces around the time of your wedding.

Because of the pandemic, we couldn't invite more than fifty guests. For some people, that may seem like a big deal. At first, I thought the same about restricting our guest list, but in the end, it was an excellent decision. During our reception, I looked around at our guests and realized I saw only people I kept in touch with. The final guest list consisted of our family and a few close friends. These were the people I truly cared about, or (as my planner says) "my ride or die" crowd.

When we sent out the notice about our dates, we asked our guests to send their negative Covid-19 test results before attending the event. We wanted to make it as safe as possible for everyone coming. Of course, that didn't completely eliminate the possibility of someone getting Covid, and I had many what-if thoughts! Those worries sometimes kept me up at night for hours. What if I tested positive and had to cancel? What if anything happened to my close friends and family members? The never-ending questions only increased my stress. In the months leading up to the wedding, I was very worried and barely wanted to leave my house to avoid getting sick.

Now, if something similar happens to you, remember not to let worry take over. Try to look at the brighter side of the situation and hope for the best. Easier said than done? Well, what else can you do? Worrying is not going to change uncontrollable events. There are many variables in situations like these, and you simply cannot control all of them. Even if it's hard, try not to worry about things that may or may not happen in the future.

To cope with my situation, I focused solely on the things that were under my control. We created a page on our website full of resources our guests could use to get tested. At that point, some guests had had their vaccinations, which helped make things a tad bit easier. We planned to have masks available and understood that some people could not make it for one reason or another. After all, safety was everybody's priority.

We encouraged people to wear masks once they arrived at the event. Some of the guests were more cautious than others. They followed all the standard procedures and maintained a safe distance on the dance floor and around other guests.

In addition to planning things on your end, keep in mind your contracts with vendors. Finding yourself in an uncertain situation requires knowing your vendors' cancellation and rescheduling policies. Also, don't forget to ask if there are restrictions on rescheduling a new date. Some vendors let you reschedule if it's within a year, and some don't transfer the deposit after a certain period has passed. Make sure you are aware of all the terms.

When you select your vendors, try to choose those who won't hesitate to reschedule and adjust according to the new norms of the current world. Wedding insurance agencies can help recover costs if a natural disaster happens and you must reschedule or do something different. My husband and I did not invest in wedding insurance, but some people find that having it helps to relieve some of the pressure and stress. If rescheduling your wedding is not a big problem, always keep this option in the back of your mind and be prepared. If there is a problem, have a backup plan ready. Perhaps a very intimate dinner or a trip with your fiancé will do. Flexibility is a great tool for stress management in difficult and uncontrollable situations.

Being a bride is an exhilarating experience but also comes with a lot of stress. Both physical and mental well-being are essential, and taking care of yourself during this time should be worked into your routine. Prioritize your own happiness and health over everything else. This day is to celebrate you and your union. Ignore the problems out of your reach, and try to take in every moment of your day because it goes by fast!

If you are considering talking with a therapist to find a healthy balance through the process of planning a wedding, don't hesitate to seek help.

One positive thing that has come out of the Covid-19 pandemic is the availability of mental health services and the significant increase in the number of people seeking help from experts. With the changing dynamics of the world, the modes of therapy have also evolved. You don't have to visit a clinic or an office to discuss your worries and concerns. Now you can receive support through phone calls, telehealth, online groups, and so on.

Therapists are professionals who strive to help you through these challenging and diffi-cult times, offering impartial and personalized advice on navigating the unknown. They provide a safe environment where people can speak freely and openly. They are there to listen, understand, advise, and guide with compassion and knowledge. Do not hesitate to seek help for your worries. Anything that troubles you, whether big or small, is worth talking about. Good coping mechanisms and support from those who love you will help you stay calm during tough days.

Chapter 5

The Dos and Don'ts

The bride and groom should remember that it is important to look back on the wedding day with happy memories. That is why so much planning is involved in the first place. Couples usually know all the major things they should or shouldn't do on their special day. Weddings are emotional events that can bring a lot of pressure and cause important tasks to be forgotten. Therefore, it's advisable to double-check everything beforehand to ensure nothing is overlooked. I almost forgot my veil before heading to the ceremony!

Review Your Timeline for Your Wedding Events

Your planner should give you a timeline

to review. Look at it carefully and make any changes if needed. Add in time for getting dressed, exchanging gifts, introductions, and transportation. Not accounting for any one of those will delay your main events. Everything is interconnected, so make sure you leave nothing out.

Prioritize the Most Important Things

Running behind or having some mishap is inevitable at a wedding. Give your most important things (for example, bridesmaids' photos) some spare time to avoid such occurrences. First, sort out what you'll prioritize. For example, some people place more importance on the event and don't care as much about photos. Instead, they want to make sure they can enjoy the live band or participate in the organized activities prepared for the guests, such as the cocktail hour. Prioritized schedules will save you time, and everything will automatically fall into place.

Start Your Preparations Early

If you think you have a lot of time, you don't! No one wants to be late for their wedding. Keep that in mind and start earlier than your set time. This will help you stay calm and give you extra time for any mishaps.

Have a Professional Do Your Makeup

Brides often hire a professional makeup artist to look their best, particularly for photographs. Although some may feel confident in their makeup application abilities, I noticed a significant difference between doing my makeup and getting it done professionally. After seeing the stunning and natural look achieved during my trial, I decided to hire a professional. However, whether or not to hire a makeup artist is ultimately a personal preference based on individual needs and skills.

Hire a Professional Photographer

If possible, I strongly suggest hiring a professional photographer for your wedding day. The day passes by quickly and is filled with a blur of emotions, fun, happiness, and love. Professional photographers have the skills to capture these fleeting moments flawlessly, resulting in beautiful memories that will last a lifetime.

Enjoy

Most importantly, enjoy every second of your day. Try to relax and embrace each moment of your day. Enjoying this day will help you tell a beautiful story.

This leads to the don'ts. Certain things

should be avoided on your big day. Below are some I learned from my experience at my wedding and being a guest at others.

Don't Try Any New Attire

Stick to what you've planned and decided on months ago. Experimenting with new dresses, veils, and shoes is risky. Don't even test out new lipsticks or face creams on that day. All those months of planning will go down the drain if any allergic reaction occurs.

Don't Forget to Take Care of Yourself

1. Don't stay up late stressing.
2. Don't skip any meals.
3. Don't start drinking early.
4. Don't be hungover.
5. Don't exercise too hard in the morning before the big day. Otherwise you'll be sore throughout the ceremony.
6. Don't take any new medications.
7. Don't forget to talk to your guests and take pictures with them.
8. Don't worry about the guests too much, and enjoy all your favorite songs.
9. Don't stay in uncomfortable clothes. Change them if you need to.
10. Don't get distracted with electronics. Ignore your phones.

Don't Schedule Hair or Spray Tan Appointments Too Close to the Wedding

Haircuts can be tricky. A man's haircut can take up to four days to look its best. Many women experience this too. It is not advisable to schedule appointments too close to the wedding as it can be risky. Services like waxing and spray tanning can also go wrong. It's best to allow these services additional time to ensure they are flawless for your big day.

Don't Make Your Guests Wait Beyond a Specific Time Limit

Take as many photos as possible before the wedding, so you don't have to spend two hours between the ceremony and reception to get the perfect shot. Most of your photographs can be taken before the start of the ceremony. Not only will you have more time at your reception, but you also won't keep your guests waiting. When you avoid this on your wedding day, your guests will be grateful.

Don't Skip the Run-Through

Rehearse everything you plan to do at the wedding. My husband didn't rehearse his vows and read only one page of them, not knowing that they were printed in two pages.

Don't Underestimate the Time It Takes to Get Ready

Hair and makeup for a group of women takes a long time. If you use a professional company, they will usually prepare a timeline to give you an idea of when you should begin getting ready. Allow at least an hour per bridesmaid per stylist if they get hair and makeup done.

Don't Forget to Eat.

Consider having some snacks beforehand to ensure you have enough energy during your wedding. With so much going on, having a full meal may be challenging. You can ask your caterers to provide appetizers or snacks for you and your spouse before the wedding begins. Eating prior will ensure you won't run on an empty stomach on your special day.

Chapter 6

Post-Wedding Blues

After the celebration and honeymoon are over, many people experience post-wedding blues. This strange feeling can be caused by a variety of factors, including adjustment in your schedule because the wedding planning is over, missing your closest friends and family, being disappointed that your honeymoon is over, or even an abstract sense of "What now?" You've just passed a huge life milestone, so you're probably nervous about all the changes ahead, whether it's a new last name, a new residence (perhaps far from friends and family), new in-laws, or a new relationship status.

It's natural to feel gloomy once all the excitement and enthusiasm around the planning has worn off. Don't worry—the post-wedding blues are real, and you're not going insane if you're upset after saying "I do." This is a special time to enjoy the beginning of your marital journey together and create memories that will last a lifetime.

As joyous and meaningful as events such as a wedding can be, the dopamine surge that often accompanies them is temporary in nature. This is because when we experience something exciting or extraordinary, the natural reaction is to become overwhelmed with emotion. The body releases a high concentration of dopamine that creates a sense of euphoria. But this rush will eventually decrease as you return to your everyday life.

So how do you cope with these feelings? You can refocus and engage in different activities to support your mental well-being. You can join a gym, start yoga, visit the local parks, and get familiar with new places. Think of things that truly please you, such as gardening, baking, or even going out for evening walks. Taking your mind off all the should-haves or could-haves can relieve you from the ongoing stress and help you focus on what you can start planning next. Maybe a new home or a baby! Some people like to give themselves a little bit of time, though. Carry on with doing those same things that used to bring you joy before all the wedding planning took over your schedule. Eventually, you will adapt or find a way back!

When you're readjusting to your new status and re-creating the new norm, the deep pit in your heart keeps returning to how exhilarating and eventful the wedding was—moments like the first time you saw your partner in their wedding outfit, the first dance, and all the fun rituals that were full of joy. But as much as it will be difficult at first, know that with a little bit of effort and perseverance, you can make this new stage of life just as meaningful.

As you were constantly planning for your wedding preparations and honeymoon, you were frequently experiencing moments of excitement. To help you adjust to this new stage, it's a good idea to schedule regular moments of joy. These don't need to be extravagant or expensive. Simple activities like game nights with friends and family or spontaneous movie marathons on weekends can bring happiness.

I hope this brief guide and my personal experiences have comforted you. Weddings can be stressful, but they are beautiful, memorable, and, most importantly, about you. Remember that your mental health is crucial, and it's normal to feel a sense of loss after transitioning into this new phase of your life. Take good care of yourself throughout the planning process and after the celebration.

Like any significant life event, the journey to your wedding is filled with ups and downs. Remember that weddings are not perfect, no matter how elaborately planned or grand they are. There will always be unexpected hiccups, but these experiences make this day uniquely yours. These real-life moments bring warmth, joy, and a bit of humor into an otherwise meticulously planned event.

Remember that love is not just about the grand gestures or the grand event. It is found in the everyday moments, in the small acts of kindness and the shared experiences that will follow your big day. The wedding is just the beginning of your journey together. The real adventure lies in the life you'll build together thereafter.

I wish you all the love and happiness in the world as you embark on this beautiful journey. May your marriage be filled with laughter, joy, and more love than you ever thought possible. And may the lessons learned from the experiences shared in this book serve as a helpful guide in planning your wedding and navigating the joys and challenges of married life.

About the Author

Claudia Marcela Chavarro graduated from the University of North Florida with a bachelor of arts in psychology. She received a master's degree in mental health counseling from Nova Southeastern University and is a licensed mental health counselor in Florida. Her areas of expertise are grief, depression, anxiety, and life adjustments.

Married in March 2021, Claudia realized how much planning goes into a wedding and how stressful it can be. Through her experience as a bride and a professional therapist, she hopes to help other brides and couples manage their big day stress-free.

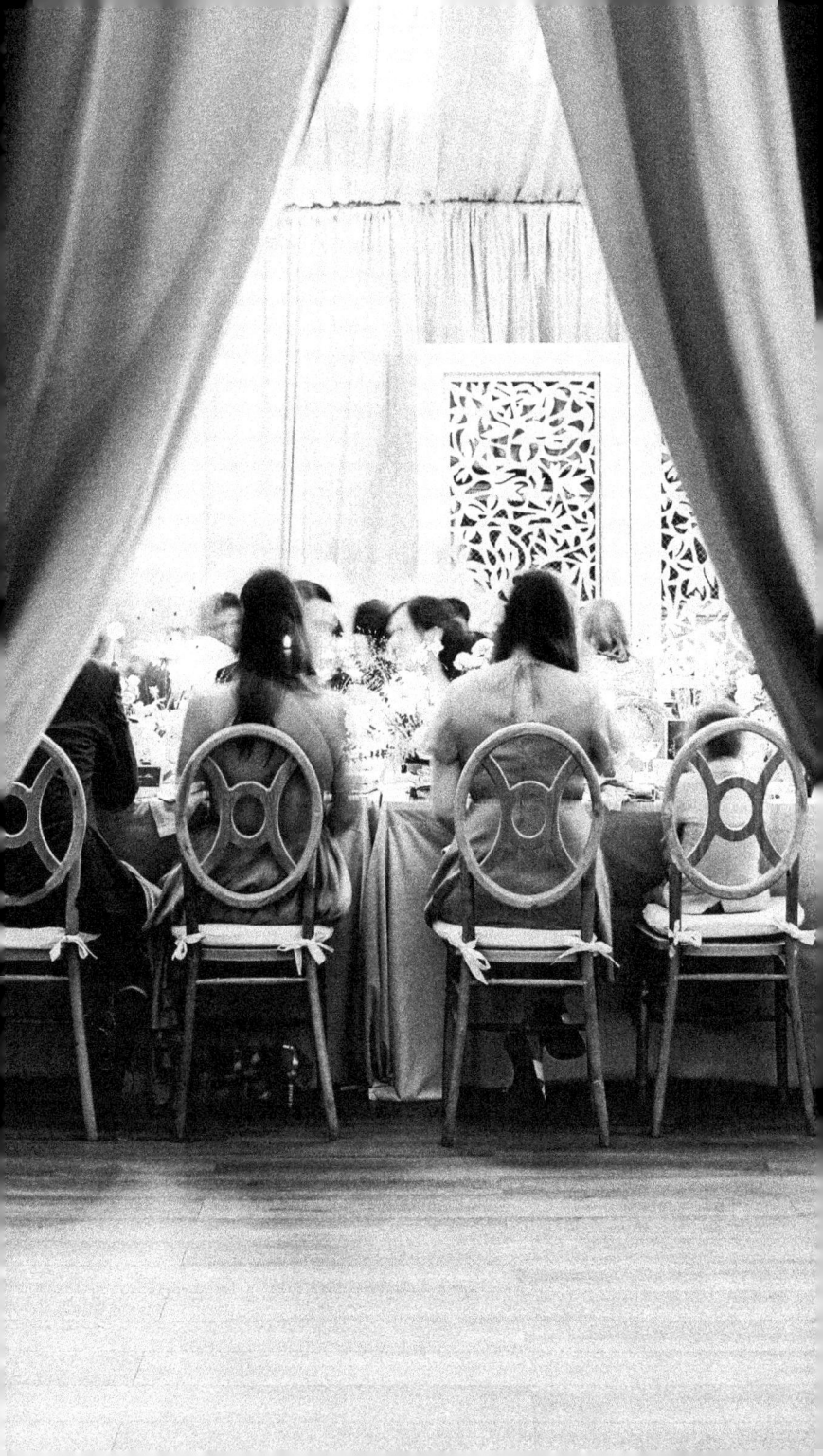

www.ingramcontent.com/pod-product-compliance
Lightning Source LLC
Chambersburg PA
CBHW070031030426
42335CB00017B/2379